The Amazing Plant-Based Breakfast Cookbook

Easy and Tasty Plant-Based Breakfast Recipes to Start Your Day and Boost Your Energy

Toby Hancock

Table of contents

Avocado Mug Bread

Preparation Time: 2 min Cooking Time: 2 min Servings: 1

Ingredients:

¼ cup Almond Flour

½ tsp Baking Powder

¼ tsp Salt

¼ cup Mashed Avocados

1 tbsp Coconut Oil

Directions:

Mix all Ingredients in a microwave-safe mug. Microwave for 90 seconds. Cool for 2 minutes.

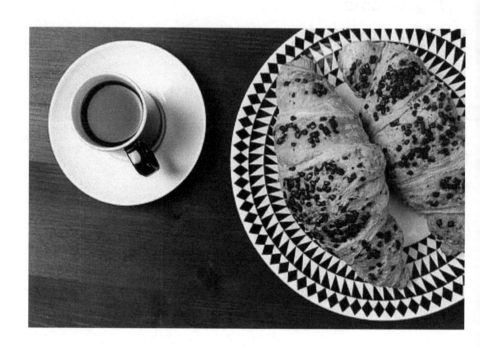

Quick Breakfast Yogurt

Preparation Time: 2 minutes Cooking Time: 8 min
Servings: 6

Ingredients:

4 cups Full-Fat Coconut Milk

2 tbsp Coconut Milk Powder

100 grams Strawberries, for serving

Directions:

Whisk together coconut milk and milk powder in a microwave safe bowl. Heat on high for 8-9 minutes. Top with fresh strawberries and choice of sweetener to serve.

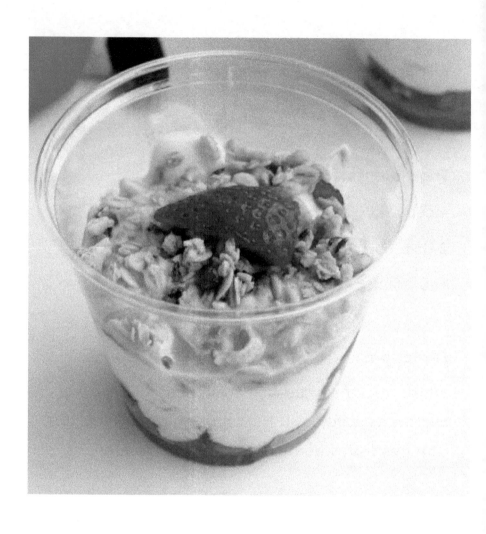

Meat-Free Breakfast Chili

Preparation Time: 10 minutes Cooking Time: 20 min

Servings: 4

Ingredients:

400 grams Textured-Vegetable Protein

¼ cup Red Kidney Beans

½ cup Canned Diced Tomatoes

1 Large Bell Pepper, diced

1 Large White Onion, diced

1 tsp Cumin Powder

1 tsp Chili Powder

1 tsp Paprika

1 tsp Garlic Powder

½ tsp Dried Oregano

2 cups Water

Directions:

Combine all Ingredients in a pot. Simmer for 20 minutes. Serve with your favorite bread or some slices of fresh avocado.

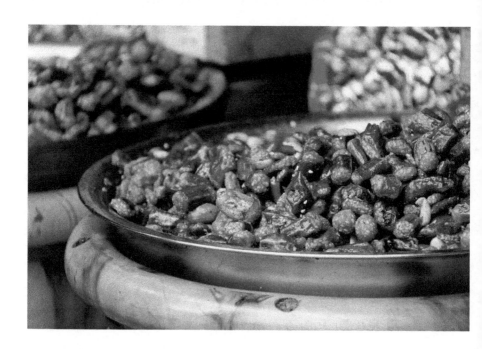

Keto Breakfast Porridge

Preparation Time: 5 minutes Cooking Time: 5 minutes
Servings: 4

Ingredients:

1 cup Flaked Coconut

½ cup Hemp Seeds

1 tbsp Coconut Flour

1 cup Water

½ cup Coconut Cream

1 tbsp Ground Cinnamon

1 tbsp Erythritol

Directions:

Combine all Ingredients in a pot. Simmer for 5 minutes, stirring continuously.

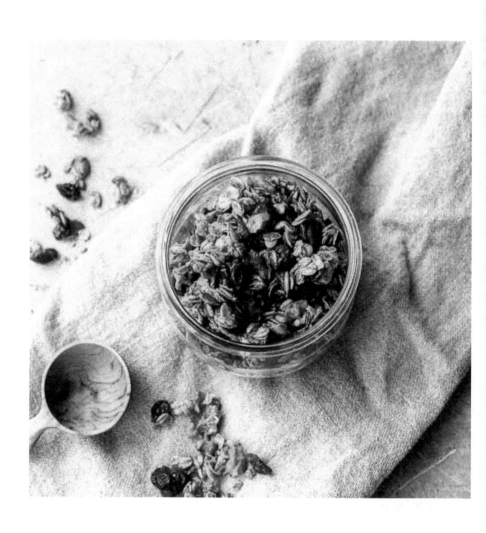

Apple Pancakes

Preparation Time: 10 minutes Cooking time: 16 minutes
Servings: 4

Ingredients:

1 and ¾ cups buckwheat flour

2 tablespoons coconut sugar

2 teaspoons baking powder

¼ teaspoon vanilla extract

2 teaspoons cinnamon powder

1 and ¼ cups almond milk

1 tablespoon flaxseed, ground mixed with

3 tablespoons water 1 cup apple, peeled, cored and chopped

A drizzle of vegetable oil

Directions:

In a bowl, mix flour with sugar, baking powder, vanilla extract and cinnamon and stir. Add flaxseed mix, milk and apple and stir well until you obtain your pancake batter. Grease your air fryer with the oil, spread ¼ of the batter, cover and cook at 360 degrees F for 5 minutes, flipping it halfway. Transfer pancake to a plate, repeat the process with the rest of the batter and serve them for breakfast. Enjoy!

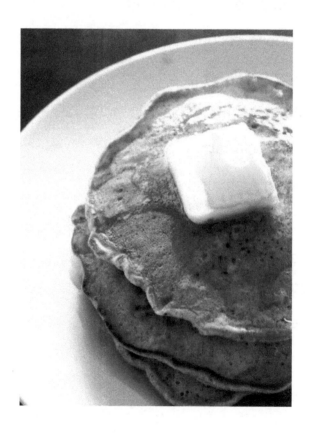

Scrambled Tofu

Preparation Time: 10 minutes Cooking time: 30 minutes

Servings: 4

Ingredients:

2 tablespoons coconut aminos

1 block firm tofu, cubed

1 teaspoon turmeric powder

2 tablespoons olive oil

½ teaspoon onion powder

½ teaspoon garlic powder

2 and ½ cup red potatoes, cubed

½ cup yellow onion, chopped

Salt and black pepper to the taste

Directions:

In a bowl, mix tofu with 1 tablespoon oil, salt, pepper, coconut aminos, garlic and onion powder, turmeric and onion and toss to coat In another bowl, mix potatoes with the rest of the oil, salt and pepper and toss. Put potatoes in preheated air fryer at 350 degrees F and bake for 15 minutes, shaking them halfway Add tofu and the marinade and bake at 350 degrees F for 15 minutes. Divide between plates and serve. Enjoy!

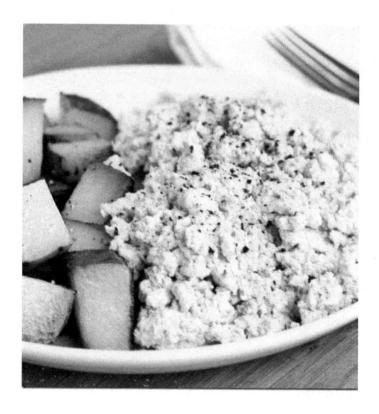

Vegan Cheese Sandwich

Preparation Time: 10 minutes Cooking time: 8 minutes
Servings: 1

Ingredients:

2 slices vegan bread

2 slices cashew cheese

2 teaspoons cashew butter

Directions:

Spread cashew butter on bread slices, add vegan cheese on one slice, top with the other, cut into halves diagonally, put in your air fryer, cover and cook at 370 degrees F for 8 minutes, flipping the sandwiches halfway. Serve them right away. Enjoy!

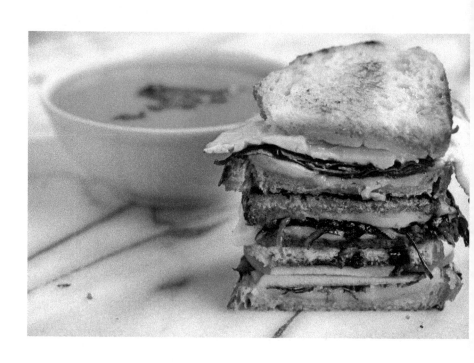

Breakfast Polenta

Preparation Time: 10 minutes Cooking time: 15 minutes

Servings: 4

Ingredients:

1 cup cornmeal

3 cups water Cooking spray

1 tablespoon coconut oil

Maple syrup for serving

Directions: Put the water for the polenta in a pot and heat up over medium heat. Add cornmeal, stir well and cook for 10 minutes. Add oil, stir again, cook for 2 minutes more, take off heat, leave aside to cool down, take spoon fools of polenta, shape balls and place them on a lined baking sheet. Grease your air fryer basket with the cooking spray , place polenta balls inside and cook them for 16 minutes at 380 degrees F flipping them halfway. Divide polenta balls between plates and serve them with some maple syrup on top. Enjoy!

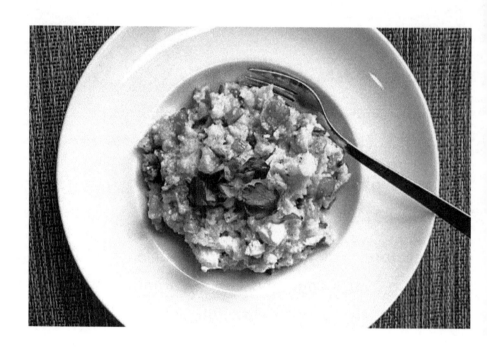

Onion and Tofu Mix

Preparation Time: 10 minutes Cooking time: 15 minutes

Servings: 2

Ingredients:

2 tablespoons flax meal mixed with

3 tablespoons water

1 yellow onion, sliced

1 teaspoon coconut aminos

Cooking spray

A pinch of black pepper

¼ cup firm tofu, cubed

Directions: In a bowl, mix flax meal with coconut aminos and black pepper and whisk well. Grease your air fryer with the cooking spray, preheat at 350 degrees F, add onion slices and cook for 10 minutes. Add flax meal and tofu, cook for 5 minutes more, divide between 2 plates and serve for breakfast. Enjoy!

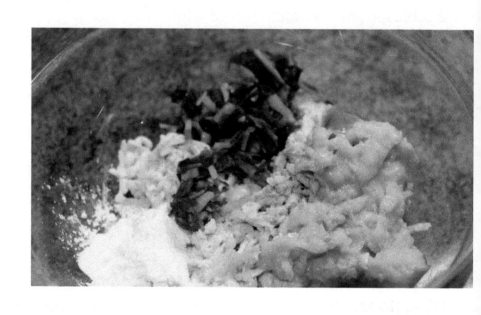

Breakfast Muffins

Preparation Time: 10 minutes Cooking time: 6 minutes
Servings: 4

Ingredients

2 cups diced banana

½ cup coconut milk, unsweetened

¼ cup coconut oil, melted

1 cup frozen sliced strawberries

2 teaspoons maple syrup

1 tablespoon ground flaxseed

⅓ cup almond flour

½ cup dates

Directions: Line muffin tins and set aside. Then add ground flax seeds, almond meal and dates into a food processor. Pulse the mixture until it becomes crumbly and then transfer to a bowl. At this point, stir in maple syrup and then press a tablespoon of crust mixture into the bottom of the muffin gently, to make the crust. Put semi-thawed strawberries in a food processor and pulse until smooth. Add in coconut and coconut milk slowly until you achieve a thick, sorbet consistency. In a bowl, add in the strawberries and gently fold in the bananas. Then sub-divide the strawberry banana mixture over the top of the crust evenly. Finally put the muffins in a freezer and let it freeze and solidify. Once frozen place in freezer bags and freeze. To serve, thaw for around 15 minutes and then serve.

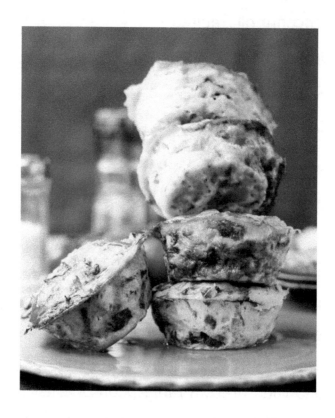

Vegan Sausage Patties

Preparation Time: 10 minutes Cooking time: 6 minutes Servings: 4

Ingredients

1 1/2 tablespoon sausage spice blend

1 cup pecans or walnuts, chopped

1 cup chickpeas, drained and rinsed

Directions: In a food processor, blend chickpeas and nuts until you have a chunky sort of paste. Plop the mixture into a bowl and stir in the spices until well incorporated. Cover the mixture and allow to set in the fridge for at least 30 minutes for flavors to blend together. In a pan placed on a stove, heat coconut or olive oil on medium-low heat. Make patties and cook them for around 10 minutes. Gently flip and cook the other side for another 10 minutes. Flip one more time and cook for 5 more minutes. Then remove from the pan and serve. You could also store them in freezer bags and freeze them to enjoy the sausages throughout the week.

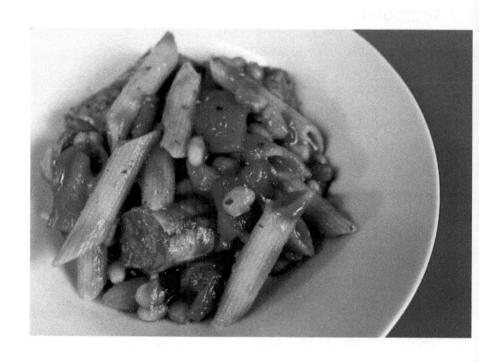

Bean Salsa Breakfast

Preparation Time: 10 minutes Cooking time: 6 minutes

Servings: 2

Ingredients

Olive oil ½ lemon

1 avocado

2 cloves of garlic

2 handfuls of spinach

1 handful of basil

6 cherry tomatoes

4 spring onions

1 can of haricot beans

Black pepper Himalayan salt

Directions: Chop the onions and the garlic and then halve the cherry tomatoes. Let 50ml water to boil in a frying pan and then steam-fry the garlic for a few seconds. Throw in the spring onions, haricot beans and the cherry tomatoes and cook until soft. Now add in the spinach and basil and cook until wilted, and season with the black pepper and Himalayan salt. Meanwhile, halve the avocado. To serve, top the bean mixture with halved avocado and lemon. You can drizzle olive oil all over the dish. Alternatively, you can freeze the bean mixture for another day. When serving, top with an avocado and some lemon.

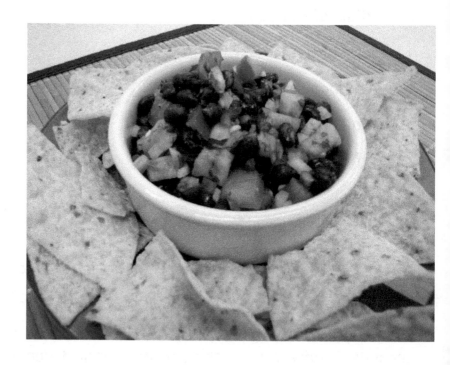

Matcha Avocado Pancakes

Preparation Time: 10 minutes Cooking Time: 5 min
Servings: 6

Ingredients:

1 cup Almond Flour

1 medium-sized Avocado, mashed

1 cup Coconut Milk

1 tbsp Matcha Powder

½ tsp Baking Soda

¼ tsp Salt

Directions:

Mix all Ingredients into a batter. Add water, a tablespoon at a time, to thin out the mixture if needed. Lightly oil a nonstick pan. Ladle approximately 1/3 cup of the batter and cook over medium heat until bubbly on the surface(about 2-3 minutes). Flip the pancake over and cook for another minute.

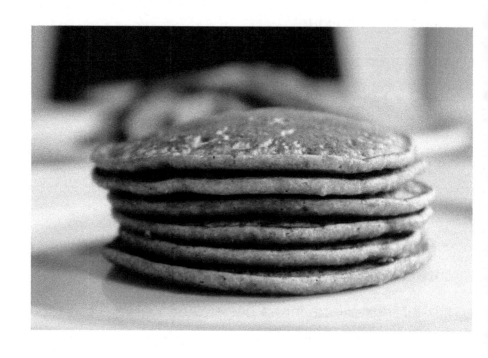

Gingerbread-Spiced Breakfast Smoothie

Preparation Time: 2 minutes Cooking Time: Servings: 2

Ingredients:

1 cup Coconut Milk

1 bag Tea

¼ tsp Cinnamon Powder

1/8 tsp Nutmeg Powder

1/8 tsp Powdered Cloves

1/3 cup Chia Seeds

2 tbsp Flax Seeds

Directions:

Put the teabag in a mug and pour in a cup of hot water. Allow to steep for a few minutes. Pour the tea into a blender together with the rest of the Ingredients. Process until smooth.

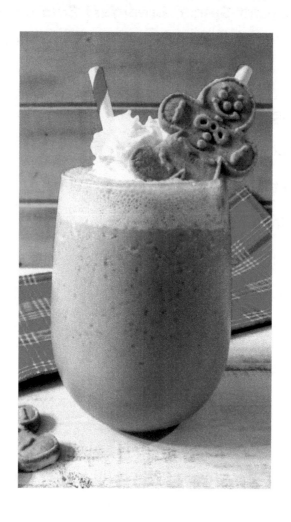

Veggie Casserole

Preparation Time: 10 minutes Cooking time: 15 minutes
Servings: 2

Ingredients:

1 yellow onion, chopped

1 teaspoon garlic, minced

1 teaspoon olive oil

1 carrot, chopped

2 celery stalks, chopped

½ cup shiitake mushrooms, chopped

½ cup red bell pepper, chopped

Salt and black pepper to the taste

1 teaspoon oregano, dried

½ teaspoon red pepper flakes

½ teaspoon cumin, ground

½ teaspoon dill, dried

7 ounces firm tofu, cubed

1 tablespoon lemon juice

2 tablespoons water

½ cup quinoa, already cooked

2 tablespoons nutritional yeast

Directions:

Heat up a pan with the oil over medium-high heat, add garlic and onion, stir and cook for 3 minutes. Add bell pepper, celery and carrot, stir and cook for 3 minutes. Add salt, pepper, mushrooms, oregano, dill, cumin and pepper flakes, stir and cook for 3 minutes more. In your food processor, mix tofu with yeast, lemon juice and water and blend well. Add quinoa and blend again. Add sautéed veggies, stir gently pour everything into your air fryer's pan and cook everything at 350 degrees F for 15 minutes. Divide your breakfast casserole between plates and serve. Enjoy!

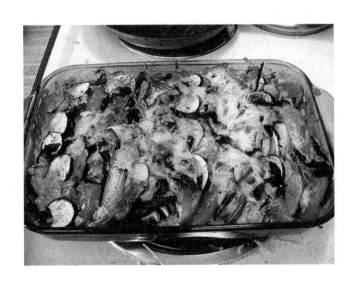

Milky Scrambled Tofu

Preparation Time: 10 minutes Cooking time: 10 minutes
Servings: 4

Ingredients:

7 ounces almond milk

2 tablespoons flax meal mixed with

2 tablespoons water

2 tablespoons firm tofu, crumbled

Cooking spray Salt and black pepper to the taste

8 cherry tomatoes, cut into halves

Directions:

In a bowl, mix flax meal with milk, salt and pepper and whisk well. Grease your air fryer with cooking spray, pour flax meal, add tofu, cook at 350 degrees F for 6 minutes, scramble them a bit and transfer to plates. Divide tomatoes on top and serve. Enjoy!

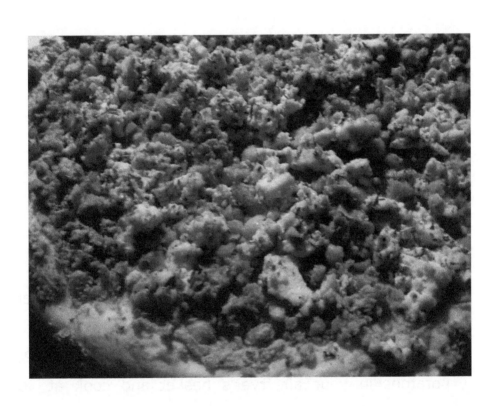

Greek Potatoes Mix

Preparation Time: 10 minutes Cooking time: 20 minutes
Servings: 4

Ingredients:

1 an ½ pounds potatoes, peeled and cubed

2 tablespoons olive oil

Salt and black pepper to the taste

1 tablespoon hot paprika ounces coconut cream

Directions:

Put potatoes in a bowl, add water to cover, leave them aside for 10 minutes, drain them, mix with half of the oil, salt, pepper and the paprika and toss them. Put potatoes in your air fryer's basket and cook at 360 degrees F for 20 minutes. In a bowl, mix coconut cream with salt, pepper and the rest of the oil and stir well. Divide potatoes between plates, add coconut cream on top and serve for breakfast Enjoy!

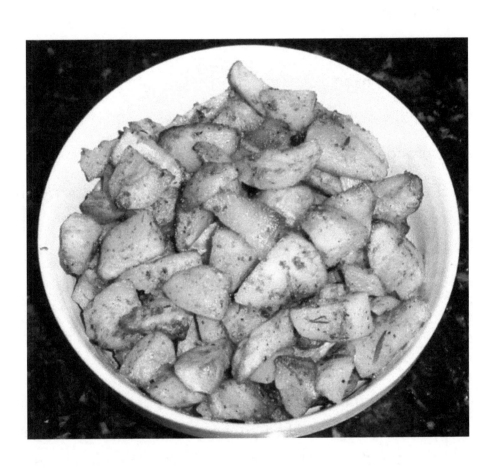

Breakfast Bell Peppers

Preparation Time: 10 minutes Cooking time: 10 minutes
Servings: 8

Ingredients:

1 yellow bell pepper, halved

1 orange bell pepper, halved

Salt and black pepper to the taste ounces firm tofu, crumbled

1 green onion, chopped

2 tablespoons oregano, chopped

Directions:

In a bowl, mix tofu with onion, salt, pepper and oregano and stir well. Place bell pepper halves in your air fryer's basket and cook at 400 degrees F for 10 minutes. Leave bell pepper halves to cool down, peel, divide tofu mix on each piece, roll, arrange on plates and serve right away for breakfast. Enjoy!

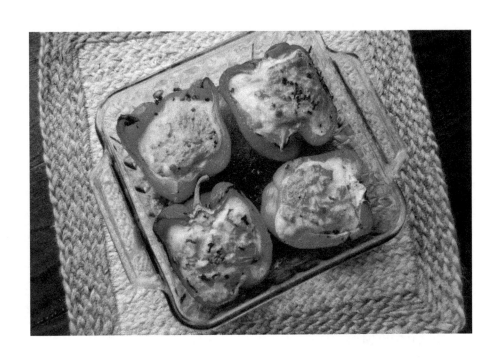

Breakfast Potatoes

Preparation time:5 minutes Cooking time: 10 minutes Servings: 6Servings: 4

Ingredients:

4 Potatoes, Peeled

1 Tablespoon Coconut Oil

½ Teaspoon Cilantro, Dried

1 Teaspoon Sea Salt

½ Teaspoon Black Pepper

1 Teaspoon Dill

1 Teaspoon Parsley

¼ Cup Water

1 Red Pepper, Chopped

1 White Onion, Chopped

Directions:

Chop your potatoes and place them in the instant pot. Add in your cilantro, coconut oi, black pepper, parsley, salt and ill. Stir and then press sauté. Cook for six minutes, and stir often to keep from burning. Add in your white onion and red pepper, and stir again. Throw in the water, and seal the lid. Cook for fifteen minutes on low pressure and then use a quick release.

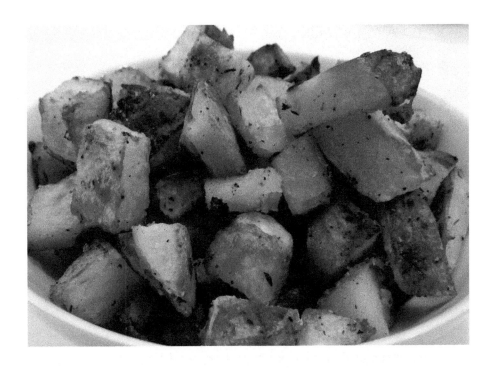

French Toast Pudding

Preparation time: 5 minutes Cooking time: 0 minutes
Servings: 5

Ingredients:

4 Bananas, Chopped

1 Cup Almond Milk

2 Tablespoons Maple Syrup

4 Slices Vegan French Bread

1 Teaspoon Vanilla Extract, Pure

1 Tablespoon Almond Butter

¼ Teaspoon Ground Cloves

1 Teaspoon Cinnamon

1 Cup Water

Directions: Pour in your water, and then get out a round pan. Chop the bread and place it on the bottom. Blend your maple syrup, chopped bananas, vanilla extract, cloves and cinnamon together until smooth, pouring it into the pan with the bread. Cover the pan with foil and make sure the edges are secure. Transfer it into the instant pot and then close your lid. Cook on high for sixteen minutes on the pudding setting. Use a quick release, and then add your almond butter in, and stir gently before serving.

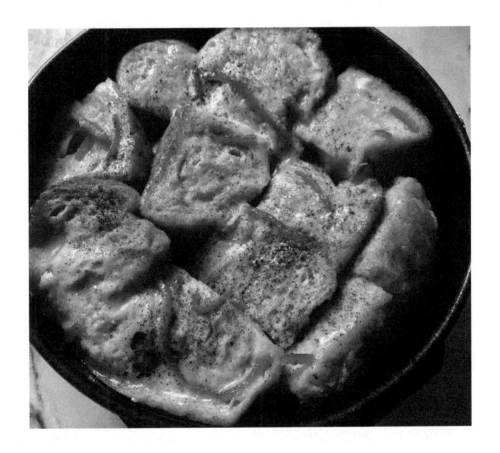

Savory Corn Pudding

Preparation time: 5 minutes Cooking time: 0 minutes Servings: 2

Ingredients:

3 Tablespoons Cornmeal

1 Cup Corn Kernels

2 Shallots, Chopped

1 Cup Coconut Milk

1 ½ Cups Water

Directions:

Press sauté, and then spritz it down with oil. Cook your shallots, and when softened add in your remaining ingredients except for the water. Pour this mixture into a baking dish before covering the dish with foil. Rinse your pot out, and then add in your water before putting your trivet in. place the baking dish on top. Seal the lid, and cook on high pressure for twenty minutes. Use a quick release to serve.

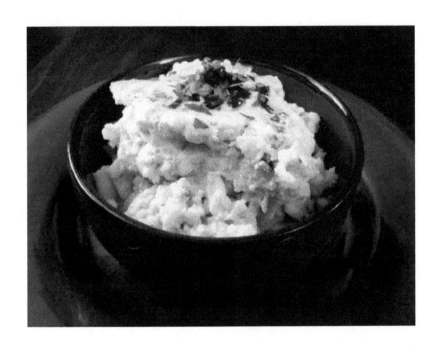

Morning Forest Maple Granola

Preparation time: 5 minutes Cooking time: 20 minutes Servings: 4 ½ cups.

Ingredients:

2 cups oats

1/3 cup pumpkin seeds

1/3 cup sunflower seeds

1/3 cup walnuts

1/3 cup unsweetened coconut flakes

¼ cup wheat germ

1 ½ tsp. cinnamon

1 cup raisins

1/3 cup maple syrup

Directions:

Begin by preheating the oven to 325 degrees Fahrenheit. Next, mix all of the above ingredients—except for the raisins and the maple syrup—together in a large bowl.

After you've mixed the ingredients well, add the maple syrup, and completely coat the other ingredients. Next, spread out this mixture on a baking sheet and bake the granola for twenty minutes, making sure to stir every four minutes or so. After twenty minutes, add the raisins and bake for an additional five minutes. Remove the baking sheet and allow the granola to cool for forty-five minutes. Enjoy!

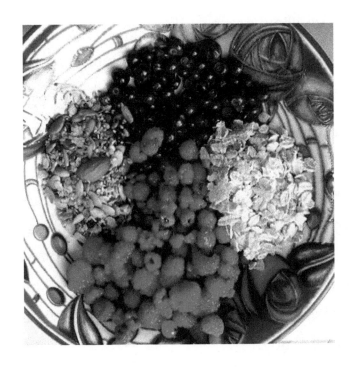

Superfood Chia Seed Breakfast Bowl

Preparation time: 5 minutes Cooking time: 35 minutes Servings: 2

Ingredients:

1/3 cup chia seeds

2 tbsp. maple syrup

2 ¼ cups soymilk

1 tsp. vanilla extract

½ cup sliced bananas or fruit of your choice

Directions:

Begin by bringing together the chia seeds, the vanilla, and the soymilk in a serving bowl. Allow this mixture to sit together for thirty minutes. Afterwards, whisk the mixture and cover it, allowing it to chill overnight in the fridge. In the morning, divide the mixture into appropriate serving sizes, and portion the banana overtop. Enjoy.

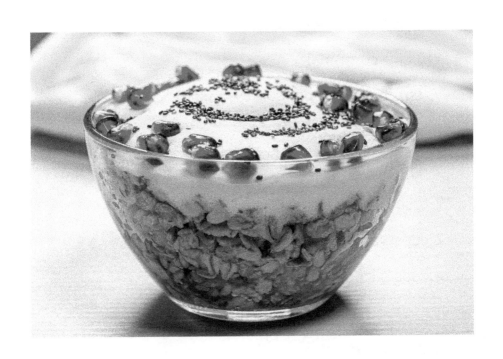

Silky Whole Wheat Strawberry Pancakes

Preparation time: 5 minutes Cooking time: 25 minutes Servings: 24 pancakes.

Ingredients:

1 ¾ cup whole wheat flour

1/3 cup cornmeal

½ tsp. baking soda

1 tsp. baking powder

½ tsp. cinnamon

2 tbsp. maple syrup

2 cups vanilla soymilk

4 cups sliced strawberries

Directions:

Begin by combining all the dry ingredients together in a mixing bowl. Stir well, and create a hole in the center of the mixture in order to pour the syrup and soymilk into it. Continue to stir, making sure not to over-stir. Next, add half of the strawberries into the mixture. Heat the skillet or the griddle, and portion just a bit of Earth Balance butter overtop. Drop little pieces of the batter onto the skillet and cook both sides of the pancakes. Keep the pancakes warm as you cook the remainder of the batter, and top the pancakes with strawberries. Enjoy.

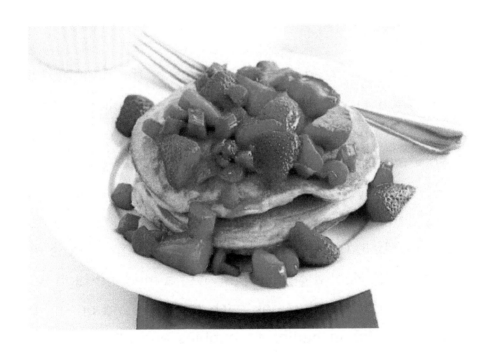

Whole Wheat Chapatti

Servings: 8 servings Preparation Time: 10 mins Cooking Time: 10 mins

Ingredients:

2½ cups whole wheat flour

¾ tsp. salt 1 cup water

Directions:

In a medium-sized bowl, mix together the flour and salt and then stir in water to form a soft, pliable dough. Scrape the dough out onto a lightly floured and clean work surface. Using your hands, knead several times to improve the dough's elasticity and smoothness. Divide the dough into 8 equal portions and roll each into a smooth ball. Using a rolling pin, roll each ball into a very thin circle. Heat a griddle pan over a medium-high heat. Do not add any oil. Cook each dough round on the pan until the dough begins to bubbles and blister, about 2 minutes. Flip over and cook until lightly brown on the other side. Serve immediately.

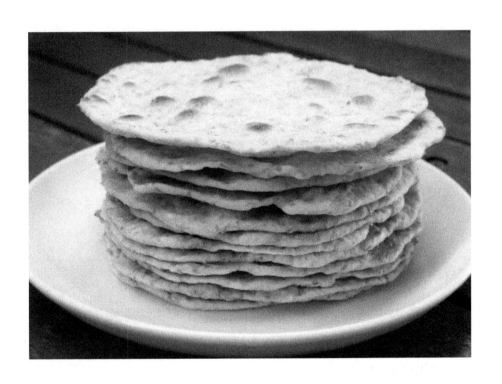

Waffles with Pumpkin & Cream Cheese

Preparation Time: 5 minutes Cooking Time: 0 minute
Serving: 1

Ingredients:

1 whole-wheat waffle

½ oz. cream cheese

1 tbsp. canned pumpkin puree

1 tsp. walnuts, toasted and chopped

Directions:

Toast the waffle. Mix the cream cheese and pumpkin.
Spread the mixture on top of the waffle. Sprinkle the
walnuts on top.

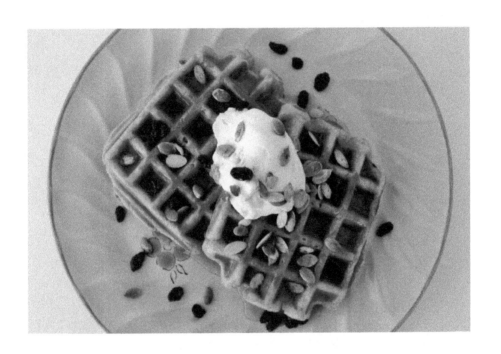

Hot Pink Smoothie

Preparation time: 5 minutes Cooking time: 0 minute Servings: 1

Ingredients:

1 clementine, peeled, segmented

1/2 frozen banana

1 small beet, peeled, chopped

1/8 teaspoon sea salt

1/2 cup raspberries

1 tablespoon chia seeds

1/4 teaspoon vanilla extract, unsweetened

2 tablespoons almond butter

1 cup almond milk, unsweetened

Directions:

Place all the ingredients in the order in a food processor or blender and then pulse for 2 to 3 minutes at high

speed until smooth. Pour the smoothie into a glass and then serve.

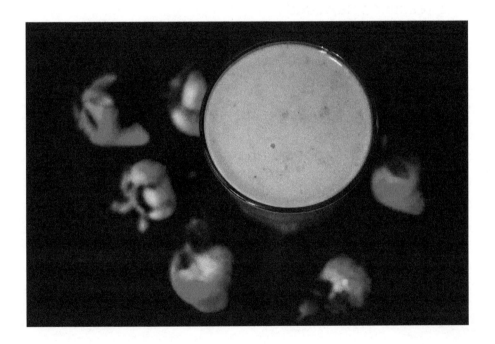

Peanut Butter Vanilla Green Shake

Preparation time: 5 minutes Cooking time: 0 minute

Servings: 1

Ingredients:

1 teaspoon flax seeds

1 frozen banana

1 cup baby spinach

1/8 teaspoon sea salt

1/2 teaspoon ground cinnamon

1/4 teaspoon vanilla extract, unsweetened

2 tablespoons peanut butter, unsweetened

1/4 cup ice

1 cup coconut milk, unsweetened

Directions:

Place all the ingredients in the order in a food processor or blender and then pulse for 2 to 3 minutes at high

speed until smooth. Pour the smoothie into a glass and then serve.

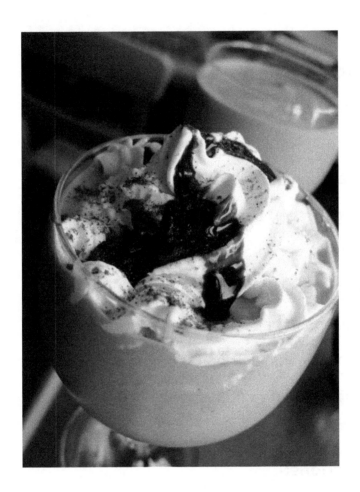

Chocolate Oat Smoothie

Preparation time: 5 minutes Cooking time: 0 minute Servings: 1

Ingredients:

¼ cup rolled oats

1 ½ tablespoon cocoa powder, unsweetened

1 teaspoon flax seeds

1 large frozen banana

1/8 teaspoon sea salt

1/8 teaspoon cinnamon

¼ teaspoon vanilla extract, unsweetened

2 tablespoons almond butter

1 cup coconut milk, unsweetened

Directions:

Place all the ingredients in the order in a food processor or blender and then pulse for 2 to 3 minutes at high

speed until smooth. Pour the smoothie into a glass and then serve.

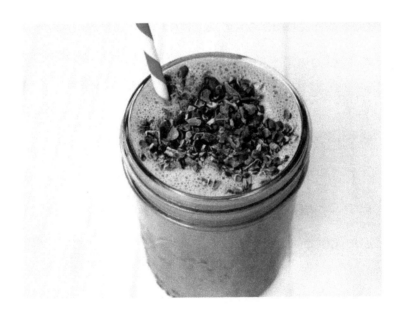

Wild Ginger Green Smoothie

Preparation time: 5 minutes Cooking time: 0 minute Servings: 1

Ingredients:

1/2 cup pineapple chunks, frozen

1/2 cup chopped kale

1/2 frozen banana

1 tablespoon lime juice

2 inches ginger, peeled, chopped

1/2 cup coconut milk, unsweetened

1/2 cup coconut water

Directions:

Place all the ingredients in the order in a food processor or blender and then pulse for 2 to 3 minutes at high speed until smooth. Pour the smoothie into a glass and then serve.

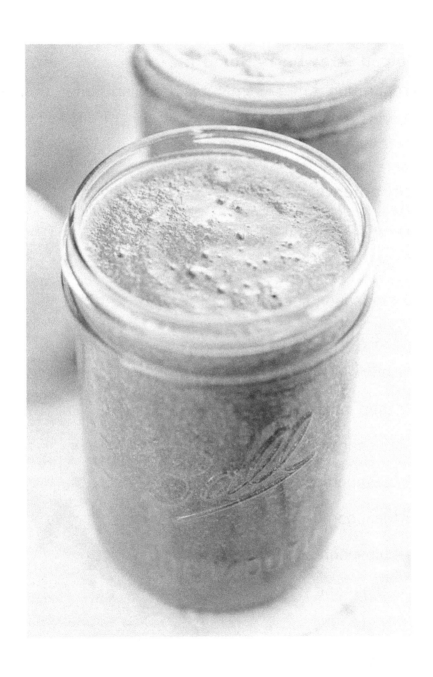

Spiced Strawberry Smoothie

Preparation time: 5 minutes Cooking time: 0 minute Servings: 1

Ingredients:

1 tablespoon goji berries, soaked

1 cup strawberries

1/8 teaspoon sea salt

1 frozen banana

1 Medjool date, pitted

1 scoop vanilla-flavored whey protein

2 tablespoons lemon juice

¼ teaspoon ground ginger

½ teaspoon ground cinnamon

1 tablespoon almond butter

1 cup almond milk, unsweetened

Directions:

Place all the ingredients in the order in a food processor or blender and then pulse for 2 to 3 minutes at high speed until smooth. Pour the smoothie into a glass and then serve.

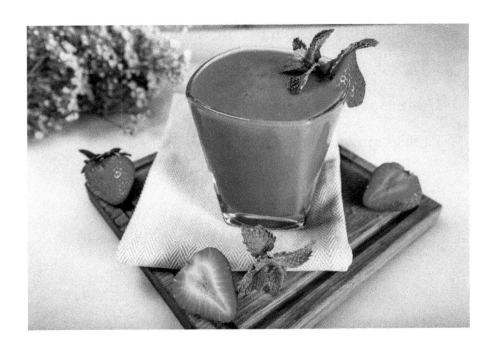

Double Chocolate Hazelnut Espresso Shake

Preparation time: 5 minutes Cooking time: 0 minute

Servings: 1

Ingredients:

1 frozen banana, sliced

1/4 cup roasted hazelnuts

4 Medjool dates, pitted, soaked

2 tablespoons cacao nibs, unsweetened

1 1/2 tablespoons cacao powder, unsweetened

1/8 teaspoon sea salt

1 teaspoon vanilla extract, unsweetened

1 cup almond milk, unsweetened

1/2 cup ice

4 ounces espresso, chilled

Directions:

Place all the ingredients in the order in a food processor or blender and then pulse for 2 to 3 minutes at high

speed until smooth. Pour the smoothie into a glass and then serve.

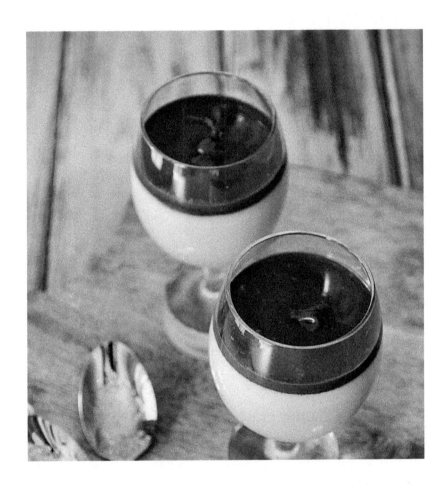

Tropical Vibes Green Smoothie

Preparation time: 5 minutes Cooking time: 0 minute
Servings: 1

Ingredients:

2 stalks of kale, ripped

1 frozen banana

1 mango, peeled, pitted, chopped

1/8 teaspoon sea salt

¼ cup of coconut yogurt

½ teaspoon vanilla extract, unsweetened

1 tablespoon ginger juice

½ cup of orange juice

½ cup of coconut water

Directions:

Place all the ingredients in the order in a food processor
or blender and then pulse for 2 to 3 minutes at high

speed until smooth. Pour the smoothie into a glass and then serve.

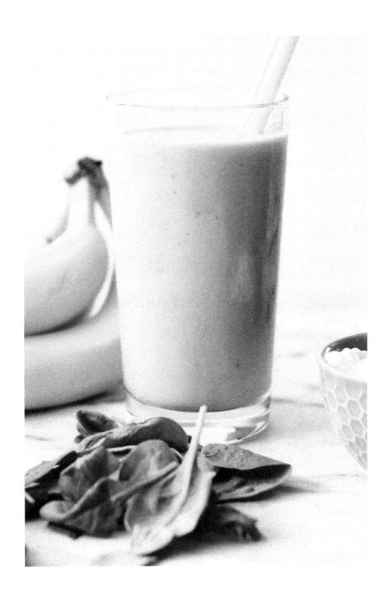

Tahini Shake with Cinnamon and Lime

Preparation time: 5 minutes Cooking time: 0 minute

Servings: 1

Ingredients:

1 frozen banana

2 tablespoons tahini

1/8 teaspoon sea salt

¾ teaspoon ground cinnamon

¼ teaspoon vanilla extract, unsweetened

2 teaspoons lime juice

1 cup almond milk, unsweetened

Directions:

Place all the ingredients in the order in a food processor or blender and then pulse for 2 to 3 minutes at high speed until smooth. Pour the smoothie into a glass and then serve.

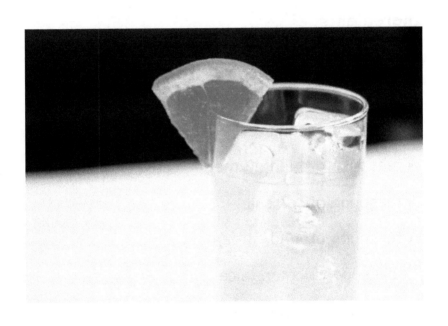

Beet and Blood Orange Smoothie

Preparation time: 5 minutes Cooking time: 0 minute
Servings: 1

Ingredients:

1 small blood orange, peeled, segmented

1 medium beet, peeled, diced

½ of frozen banana

⅛ teaspoon ground nutmeg

¼ teaspoon of sea salt

¼ teaspoon ground cardamom

2 tablespoons lemon juice

½ teaspoon ground cinnamon

1 tablespoon almond butter

1 cup of coconut milk, unsweetened

Directions:

Place all the ingredients in the order in a food processor
or blender and then pulse for 2 to 3 minutes at high

speed until smooth. Pour the smoothie into a glass and then serve.

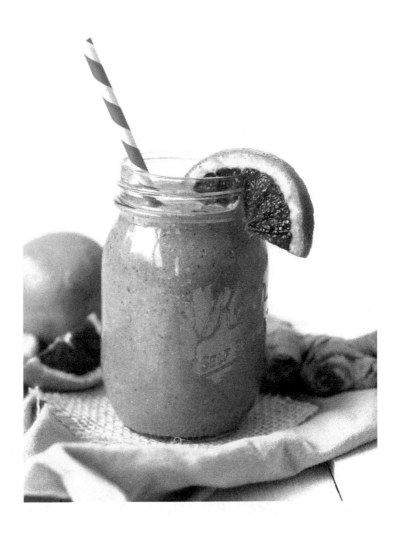

Strawberry and Raspberry Smoothie

Preparation time: 5 minutes Cooking time: 0 minute Servings: 1

Ingredients:

1 cup frozen raspberries

3 Medjool dates, pitted

1 cup spinach

1 cup of frozen strawberries

1 scoop of vanilla protein powder

2 tablespoons almond butter

1 3/4 cups almond milk

Directions:

Place all the ingredients in the order in a food processor or blender and then pulse for 2 to 3 minutes at high speed until smooth. Pour the smoothie into a glass and then serve

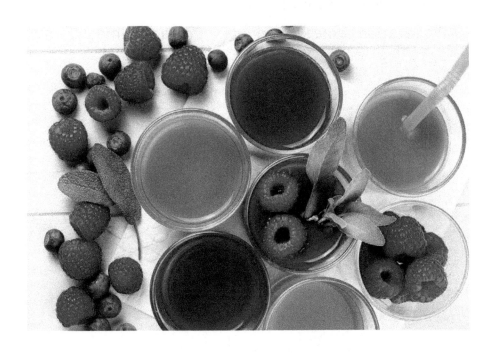

Chocolate Banana Smoothie

Preparation time: 5 minutes Cooking time: 0 minute Servings: 1

Ingredients:

1 cup spinach 1 frozen banana

1 tablespoon chia seeds

2 tablespoon cacao powder, unsweetened

1 tablespoon ground flax seeds

1/2 teaspoon sea salt

1 teaspoon maca powder

1 scoop of vanilla protein powder

1 1/2 cups almond milk, unsweetened

Directions:

Place all the ingredients in the order in a food processor or blender and then pulse for 2 to 3 minutes at high

speed until smooth. Pour the smoothie into a glass and then serve.

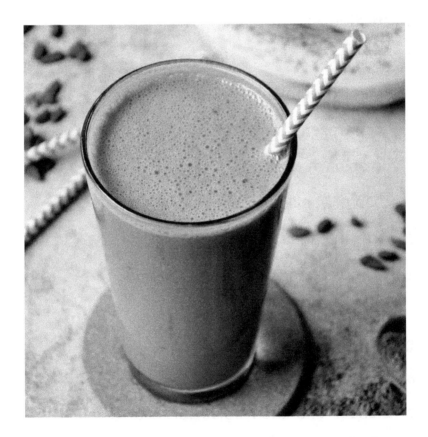

Mixed Berry Smoothie

Preparation time: 5 minutes Cooking time: 0 minute Servings: 1

Ingredients:

1/2 cup frozen raspberries

1/2 cup frozen blueberries

1/2 cup frozen strawberries

1 cup spinach

1 scoop of vanilla protein powder

1/2 frozen banana

1 3/4 cups almond milk, unsweetened

Directions:

Place all the ingredients in the order in a food processor or blender and then pulse for 2 to 3 minutes at high speed until smooth. Pour the smoothie into a glass and then serve.

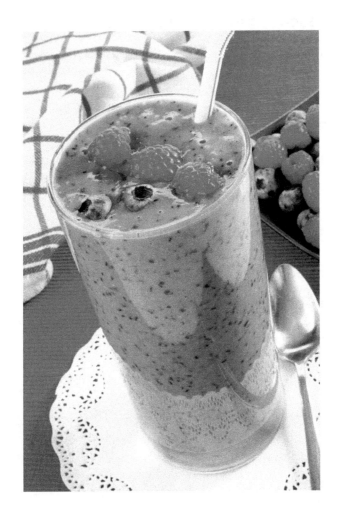

Mango and Pineapple Smoothie

Preparation time: 5 minutes Cooking time: 0 minute Servings: 1

Ingredients:

3/4 cup mango chunks, frozen

1 cup sliced cucumber

1 cup pineapple chunks, frozen

2 cups fresh spinach

1 scoop of vanilla protein powder

1 teaspoon moringa powder

1 teaspoon pure vanilla extract, unsweetened

1 2/3 cup almond milk, unsweetened

Directions:

Place all the ingredients in the order in a food processor or blender and then pulse for 2 to 3 minutes at high

speed until smooth. Pour the smoothie into a glass and then serve.

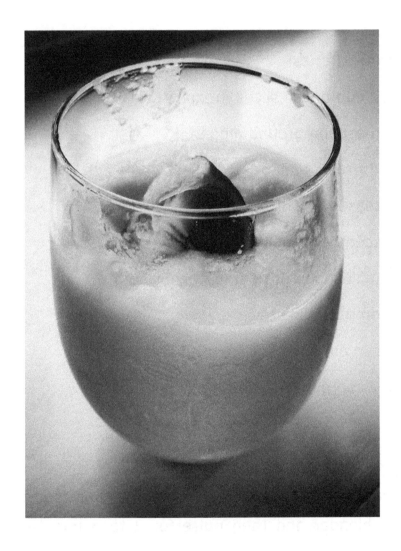

Peanut Butter and Pumpkin Smoothie

Preparation time: 5 minutes Cooking time: 0 minute

Servings: 1

Ingredients:

1/2 cup peach slices, frozen

2 teaspoon ground ginger

1/2 frozen banana

1 teaspoon cinnamon

1 scoop of vanilla protein powder

4 tablespoon powdered peanut butter

5 drops liquid stevia

1 cup almond milk, unsweetened

1/2 cup pumpkin puree

Directions:

Place all the ingredients in the order in a food processor or blender and then pulse for 2 to 3 minutes at high

speed until smooth. Pour the smoothie into a glass and then serve.

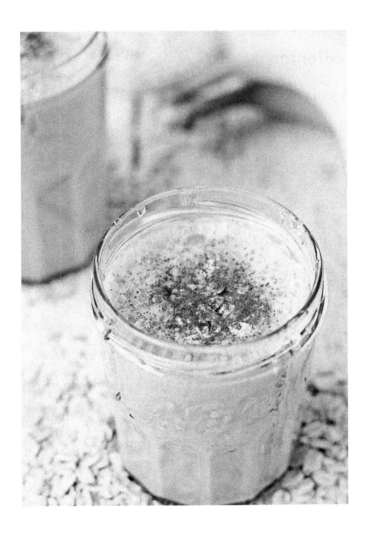

Blueberry and Sweet Potato Smoothie

Preparation time: 5 minutes Cooking time: 0 minute Servings: 1

Ingredients:

1 1/4 cup frozen blueberries

1/2 cup frozen sweet potato, cooked

1/8 teaspoon sea salt

1 tablespoon cacao powder

1 scoop of chocolate protein powder

1 cup almond milk

Directions:

Place all the ingredients in the order in a food processor or blender and then pulse for 2 to 3 minutes at high speed until smooth. Pour the smoothie into a glass and then serve.

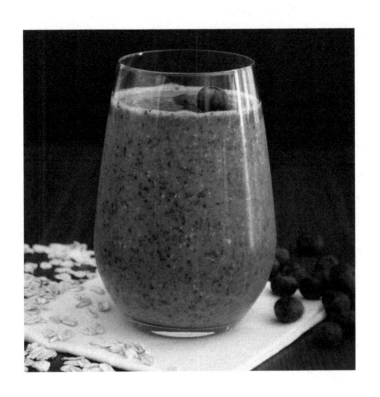

Breakfast Sandwich

Preparation time: 5 minutes Cooking time: 6 minutes Servings: 4

Ingredients:

¼ of a medium avocado, sliced

1 vegan sausage patty

2 teaspoon olive oil

1 cup kale

1/8 teaspoon salt

1/8 teaspoon black pepper

1 Tablespoon pepitas

1 English muffin, halved, toasted

For the Sauce:

1 teaspoon jalapeno, chopped

1/8 teaspoon smoky paprika

1 tablespoon mayonnaise, vegan

Directions:

Take a saute pan, place it over medium heat, add oil and when hot, add the patty and cook for 2 minutes. Then slip the patty, push it to one side of the pan, add kale and pepitas to the other side, season with black pepper and salt, and cook for 2 to 3 minutes until kale has softened. When done, remove the pan from heat and prepare the sauce by whisking its ingredients until combined. Assemble the sandwich and for this, spread mayonnaise on the inside of muffin, top with avocado slices and patty, and then top with kale and pepitas. Serve straight.

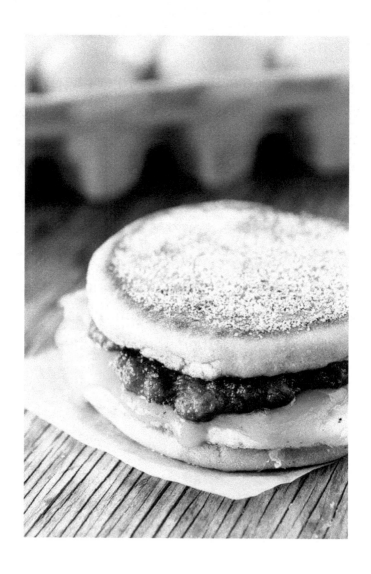

Potato Skillet Breakfast

Preparation time: 5 minutes Cooking time: 15 minutes
Servings: 5

Ingredients:

1 ½ cup cooked black beans

1 1/4 pounds potatoes, diced

12 ounces spinach, destemmed

1 1/4 pounds red potatoes, diced

2 small avocados, sliced, for topping

1 medium green bell pepper, diced

1 jalapeno, minced

1 large white onion, diced

1 medium red bell pepper, diced

3 cloves of garlic, minced

1/2 teaspoon red chili powder

1/4 teaspoon salt

1 teaspoon cumin

1 tablespoon canola oil

Directions:

Switch on the oven, then set it to 425 degrees F and let it preheat. Meanwhile, take a skillet pan, place it over medium heat, add oil and when hot, add potatoes, season with salt, chili powder, and cumin, stir until mixed and cook for 2 minutes. Transfer pan into the oven and roast potatoes for 20 minutes until cooked, stirring halfway through. Then add remaining onion, bell peppers, garlic, and jalapeno, continue roasting for another 15 minutes, stirring halfway, and remove the pan from heat. Transfer pan over medium heat, cook for 5 to 10 minutes until potatoes are thoroughly cooked, then stir spinach and beans and cook for 3 minutes until spinach leaves have wilted. When done, top the skillet with cilantro and avocado and then serve.

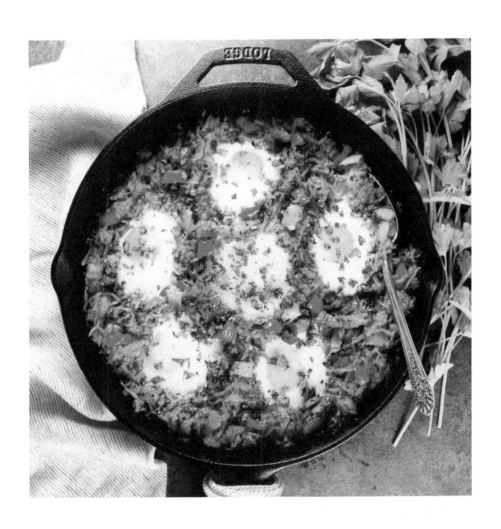

Peanut Butter and Banana Bread Granola

Preparation time: 10 minutes Cooking time: 32 minutes
Servings: 6

Ingredients:

1/2 cup Quinoa

1/2 cup mashed banana

3 cup rolled oats, old-fashioned

1 cup banana chips, crushed

1 cup peanuts, salted

1 teaspoon. salt

1 teaspoon. cinnamon

1/4 cup brown sugar

1/4 cup honey

2 teaspoon. vanilla extract, unsweetened

1/3 cup peanut butter

6 tablespoon. unsalted butter

Directions:

Switch on the oven, then set it to 325 degrees F and let it preheat. Meanwhile, take two rimmed baking sheets, line them with parchment sheets, and set aside until required. Place oats in a bowl, add quinoa, banana chips, cinnamon, salt, and sugar and stir until combined. Take a small saucepan, place it over medium-low heat, add butter and honey and cook for 4 minutes until melted, stirring frequently. Then remove the pan from heat, add banana and vanilla, stir until mixed, then spoon the mixture into the oat mixture and stir until incorporated. Distribute granola evenly between two baking sheets, spread evenly, and then bake for 25 minutes until golden brown, rotating the sheets halfway. When done, transfer baking sheets on wire racks, cool the granola, then break it into pieces and serve. Serve straight away.

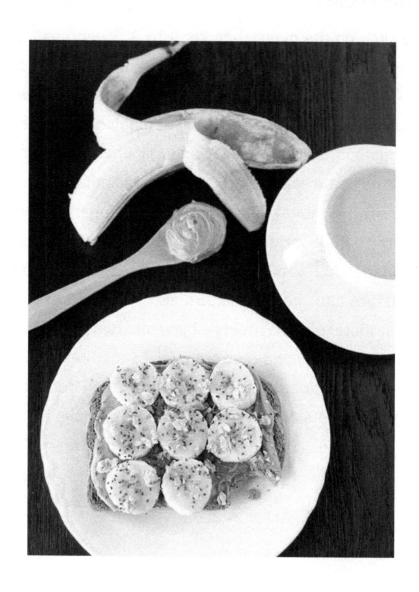

Chickpea Flour Omelet

Preparation time: 5 minutes Cooking time: 12 minutes Servings: 1

Ingredients:

1/4 cup chickpea flour

1/2 teaspoon chopped chives

½ cup spinach, chopped

1/4 teaspoon turmeric

1/4 teaspoon garlic powder

1/8 teaspoon ground black pepper

1/2 teaspoon baking power

1 tablespoon nutritional yeast

1/2 teaspoon vegan egg

1/4 cup and

1 tablespoon water

Directions:

Take a bowl, place all the ingredients in it, except for spinach, whisk until combined and let it stand for 5 minutes. Then take a skillet pan, place it over low heat, grease it with oil and when hot, pour in prepared and cook for 3 minutes until edges are dry. Then top half of the omelet with spinach, fold with the other half and continue cooking for 2 minutes. Slide omelet to a plate and serve with ketchup.

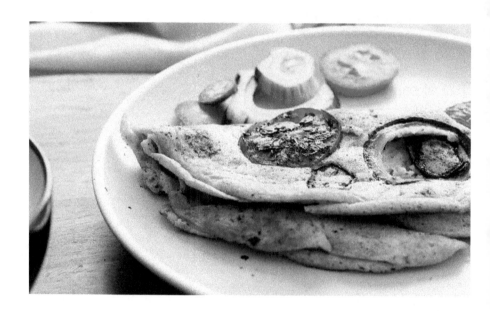

Vegetarian Breakfast Casserole

Preparation time: 10 minutes Cooking time: 35 minutes

Servings: 4

Ingredients:

5 medium potatoes, about 22 ounces, boiled

10 ounces silken tofu

5 ounces tempeh, cubed

1 tablespoon chives, cut into rings

1 medium white onion, peeled chopped

¾ teaspoon ground black pepper

1 ½ teaspoon salt

1 teaspoon turmeric

2 1/2 teaspoons paprika powder

1 1/2 tablespoons olive oil

1 tablespoon corn starch

1 teaspoon soy sauce

1 tablespoon barbecue sauce

1/2 teaspoon liquid smoke

1/2 cup vegan cheese

Directions:

Switch on the oven, then set it to 350 degrees F and let it preheat. Meanwhile, peel the boiled potatoes, then cut them into cubes and set aside until required. Prepare tempeh and for this, take a skillet pan, place it over medium heat, add half of the oil, and when hot, add half of the onion and cook for 1 minute. Then add tempeh pieces, season with 1 teaspoon paprika, add soy sauce, liquid smoke and BBQ sauce, season with salt and black pepper and cook tempeh for 5 minutes, set aside until required. Take a large skillet pan, place it over medium heat, add remaining oil and onion and cook for 2 minutes until beginning to soften. Then add potatoes, season with ½ teaspoon paprika, salt, and black pepper to taste and cook for 5 minutes until crispy, set aside until required. Take a medium bowl, place tofu in it, then add remaining ingredients and whisk until smooth. Take a casserole dish, place potatoes and tempeh in it, top with tofu mixture, sprinkle some more cheese, and bake for 20 minutes until done. Serve straight away.

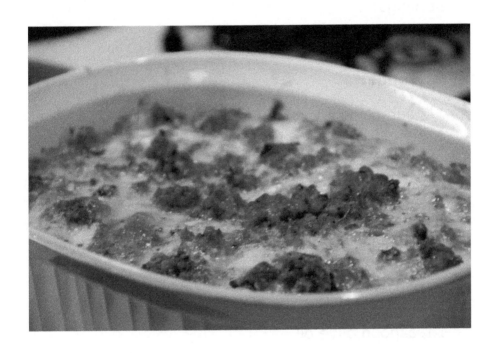

Chickpea and Zucchini Scramble

Preparation time: 5 minutes Cooking time: 20 minutes Servings: 2

Ingredients:

1/2 cup diced zucchini

1/4 cup chopped onions

¼ teaspoon ground black pepper

1 tablespoon thyme, chopped

½ teaspoon salt

1/2 cup chickpea flour

1 teaspoon olive oil

1/2 cup vegetable broth

Directions:

Take a medium bowl, add chickpea flour and then whisk in broth until smooth. Take a medium skillet pan, place it over medium-high heat, add oil and when hot, add onion and cook for 5 minutes. Add zucchini, continue cooking for 5 minutes until vegetables begin to brown, and then season vegetables with black pepper, salt, and thyme and stir until mixed. Then stir in chickpea flour mixture and cook for 5 to 10 minutes until cooked and mixture is no longer wet Serve straight away.

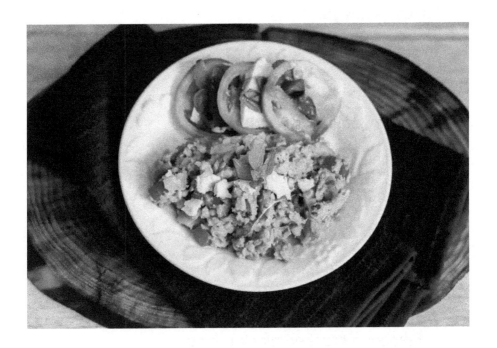

Breakfast Tacos

Preparation time: 15 minutes Cooking time: 0 minute Servings: 4

Ingredients:

For The Filling:

12 ounces of cooked black bean and tofu scramble

For the Mango

Pineapple Salsa:

1/3 cup diced tomatoes

1 medium shallot, peeled, diced

½ cup diced mango

1 jalapeno, deseeded, diced

2 teaspoon minced garlic

½ cup diced pineapple

1 tablespoon cilantro

¼ teaspoon cracked black pepper

¼ teaspoon salt

2 tablespoons lime juice

For The Tacos:

1 avocado, pitted, diced

4 small tortillas, warmed Chopped cilantro for garnish

Directions:

Prepare salsa and for this, place all its ingredients in a bowl and stir until mixed. Then prepare tofu scramble, distribute it evenly between tortillas and top evenly with prepared salsa and avocado. Garnish with cilantro and serve.

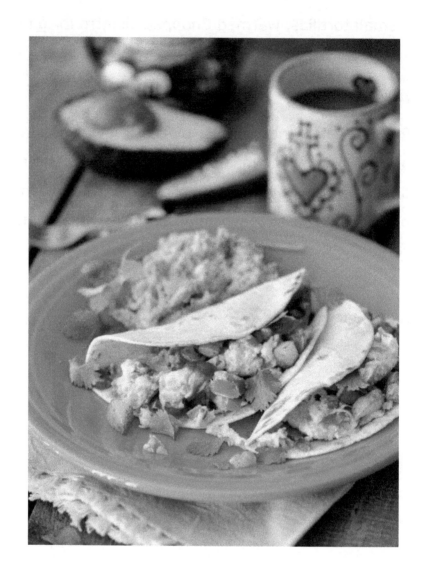

Fig Oatmeal Bake

Preparation time: 5 minutes Cooking time: 15 minutes

Servings: 4

Ingredients:

2 fresh figs, sliced

5 dried figs, chopped

4 tablespoons chopped walnuts

1 ½ cups oats

1 teaspoon cinnamon

2 tablespoons agave syrup

1 teaspoon baking powder

2 tablespoons unsalted butter, melted

3 tablespoons flaxseed egg

¾ cup of coconut milk

Directions:

Switch on the oven, then set it to 350 degrees F and let it preheat. Meanwhile, take a bowl, place all the ingredients in it, except for fresh figs and stir until combined. Take an 8-inch square pan, line it with parchment sheet, spoon in the prepared mixture, top with fig slices, and bake for 30 minutes until cooked and set. Serve straight away.

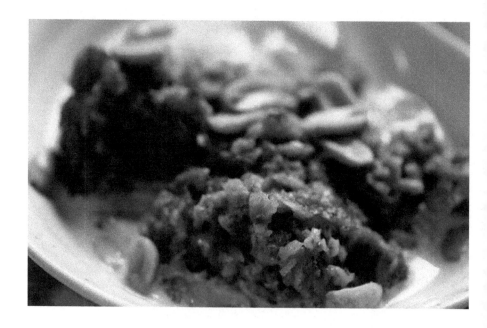

Vegan Fried Egg

Preparation time: 5 minutes Cooking time: 8 minutes
Servings: 4

Ingredients:

1 block of firm tofu, firm, pressed, drained

½ teaspoon ground black pepper

½ teaspoon salt

1 tablespoon vegan butter

1 cup vegan toast dipping sauce

Directions:

Cut tofu into four slices, and then shape them into a rough circle by using a cookie cutter. Take a frying pan, place it over medium heat, add butter and when it melts, add prepared tofu slices in a single layer and cook for 3 minutes per side until light brown. Transfer tofu to serving dishes, make a small hole in the middle of tofu by using a small cookie cutter and fill the hole with dipping sauce. Garnish eggs with black pepper and sauce and then serve.

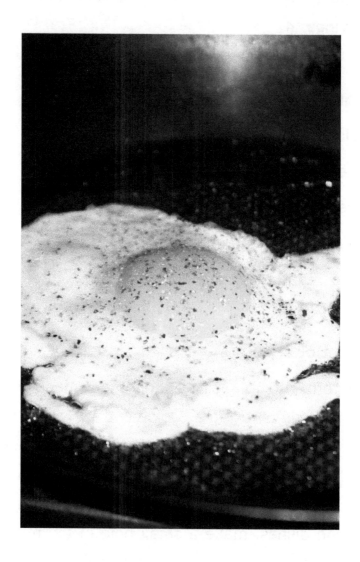

Lightning Source UK Ltd.
Milton Keynes UK
UKHW020659240521
384264UK00005B/109